Complete Metabolic Confusion Diet Guide for Endomorph Women

Empower Your Endomorph Journey, Boost Your Metabolism, Revitalize Your Body, and Embrace Wellness with Delicious Recipes and Strategic Lifestyle Changes.

Donna Johnson

TABLE OF CONTENTS

1. INTRODUCTION TO METABOLIC CONFUSION

What is Metabolic Confusion?

Metabolic Confusion is a deliberate eating method that tries to avoid metabolic standstill, a typical mistake made by dieters who follow standard diets. It is not simply a diet. Essentially, this approach entails adjusting one's daily or weekly consumption of calories and macronutrients. The word "confusion" comes from the belief that this variation keeps the metabolism busy and guessing.

Metabolic Confusion is more dynamic than strict diet regimens that dictate a certain amount of calories to be consumed. It fluctuates between times when you consume more and less calories. The body gets enough of energy during high-calorie times, which may raise metabolic rate. On the other hand, the body is urged to use fat reserves as energy during low-calorie periods, which aids in weight reduction.

The body's built-in adaptive systems provide the foundation for the reasoning behind Metabolic Confusion. Generally, the body slows down the metabolism to preserve energy when the calorie intake is continuously low, as in traditional diets. This adaptive reaction may cause weight reduction to plateau, making it difficult to go forward.

The goal of Metabolic Confusion is to avoid this delay in metabolism. It attempts to maintain the metabolism active and prevent it from slowing down by varying the amount of calories consumed on a regular basis. This strategy is said to increase fat burning, increase metabolic flexibility, and maybe result in weight reduction that is more long-lasting.

This method may be especially helpful for endomorph women, who typically battle with a naturally sluggish metabolism. Endomorphs often have a greater body fat percentage, thus they can have more difficulty losing weight with traditional steady-state diets that limit their calorie intake. With its fluctuating calorie intake, metabolic confusion may be a useful tactic to speed up their metabolism and help them control their weight more successfully.

The fundamental ideas of Metabolic Confusion include switching between varying calorie and macronutrient intakes. Depending on personal objectives and reactions, these variations might have a daily, weekly, or even bi-weekly schedule. The goal of the high-calorie days is to properly nourish the body with nutrient-dense meals rather than merely ingesting more calories. Conversely, low-calorie days place more of an emphasis on calorie restriction while still requiring a macronutrient-balanced diet.

Understanding Your Metabolism

The intricate web of biochemical activities that take place within our bodies is referred to as metabolism. It includes turning food and liquids into energy, which is needed for a number of internal processes, such as blood circulation, respiration, hormone regulation, and cell repair. Since metabolism is essential to how our bodies consume and store energy, it is often brought up in discussions about weight control.

Catabolism and anabolism are the two main processes that make up metabolism. While anabolism utilizes this energy to make new biological molecules and repair and rebuild tissues, catabolism breaks down molecules to produce energy. The way our bodies utilize the energy from meals depends on the balance between these two processes.

The pace at which your body burns calories is known as your metabolic rate. It is impacted by many factors:

Basal Metabolic Rate (BMR): The energy used up while the body is at rest. Age, sex, genetics, and body composition are some of the elements that influence it.

Physical Activity: Exercising and going about your regular business help you burn more calories than your body mass index.

The energy needed for nutritional digestion, absorption, and assimilation is known as the "thermic effect of food" (TEF).

Endomorphs often have slower metabolisms due to their increased body fat percentage and inclination to conserve energy. This may make losing weight more difficult. In particular, insulin resistance and hormonal balance might have an additional impact on endomorph women's metabolism.

Knowing your metabolic rate alone won't help you understand your metabolic health. It includes being aware of how various diets, stress levels, sleep schedules, and physical exercise affect your body. Hormonal balance, energy levels, and general well-being are all strongly correlated with metabolic health.

The body's capacity to effectively adjust to different metabolic demands, such as alternating between burning fats and carbs for energy, is known as metabolic flexibility. One of the main ideas of the Metabolic Confusion method is that weight control and energy usage may both be improved by increasing metabolic flexibility.

It's a good idea to evaluate your metabolic health before starting the Metabolic Confusion diet. Medical examinations, knowledge of body composition, and monitoring your body's response to various diets and exercise regimens may all help achieve this.

Everybody has a different metabolism. As such, a one-size-fits-all strategy is ineffective. Gaining an understanding of your metabolism will enable you to customize the Metabolic Confusion diet to your unique requirements, increasing its efficacy as a weight-management and health-improving strategy.

Why This Diet is tailored for Endomorph Women

Understanding the traits of the endomorph body type is crucial in order to appreciate why the Metabolic Confusion diet is appropriate for endomorph women. Generally speaking, endomorphs have a fuller build, a greater body fat percentage, and an inclination to put on weight quickly. Their metabolisms are often slower than average, which may make controlling their weight more difficult.

Women who are endomorphic have unique metabolic obstacles that may impede their attempts to reduce weight. Among them are:

Slower Metabolic Rate: Compared to other body types, endomorphs often have a slower basal metabolic rate (BMR), which results in reduced resting-state calorie expenditure.

Additionally, they could be more vulnerable to insulin resistance, which might make it harder for them to control their blood sugar levels and perhaps result in weight gain.

Endomorphs have a tendency to store energy more easily as fat, particularly around the abdomen.

In light of these difficulties, the Metabolic Confusion diet is designed to specifically cater to the requirements of endomorphic women by:

Improving Metabolic Flexibility: This diet may increase metabolism by helping the body become more adept at switching between utilizing fats and carbohydrates for energy. It does this by altering the amount of calories consumed.

Avoiding Metabolic Adaptation: By alternating days with high and low calories, you may keep your body from becoming used to a certain calorie intake, which can help you avoid reaching weight loss plateaus.

Increasing Insulin Sensitivity: Altering your diet on a regular basis may help you become more sensitive to insulin and better at controlling your blood sugar levels.

Benefits of the Metabolic Confusion diet for endomorphic women include:

Long-Term and greater Sustainable Weight reduction: This diet encourages greater long-term and sustainable weight reduction by avoiding metabolic slowing.

Enhanced Energy: Changing up your food will help you better control your energy levels and prevent the exhaustion that comes with following a tight diet plan.

Enhanced Nutrient consumption: For general health and well-being, a balanced nutrient consumption is encouraged by this diet.

Although the fundamentals of Metabolic Confusion remain the same, customization of the program is both possible and desirable. When following this diet, endomorphic women should take into account things like their level of exercise, way of life, and unique metabolic reactions. To meet unique demands and objectives, customization may include modifying the duration of high- and low-calorie intervals, the precise calorie intake, and the macronutrient composition.

The Metabolic Confusion diet should be combined with regular exercise and a healthy lifestyle for best results. Strength training helps endomorph women gain lean muscle mass; cardiovascular workouts help them become more fit overall and help them lose fat.

2. ENDOMORPH BODY TYPE EXPLAINED

Identifying Your Body Type

Ectomorph, mesomorph, and endomorph body types are the three basic categories used to describe body types in the context of exercise and nutrition. Every variety has unique physical attributes and metabolic inclinations.

Ectomorphs usually have a long, slender build and have trouble putting on weight or muscle.

Mesomorphs have a higher metabolism, increased muscular mass, more sensitive muscle fibers.

The typical characteristics of endomorphs are a slower metabolism, less defined muscles, and a larger proportion of body fat.

Knowing these categories is about identifying and working with your body's innate inclinations, not about labeling or restricting yourself.

The tendency to accumulate fat is the main characteristic of the endomorph body type. Typical characteristics consist of:

A more rounded physique with a greater proportion of body fat.

A slower metabolism, which makes weight gain simple and weight loss difficult.

A more rounded, soft-looking body with fewer pronounced muscles.

It's crucial to remember that each individual might have these traits differently, and many individuals may discover that they have traits with many body types.

There is more to determining your body type than merely glancing in the mirror. It involves being aware of how your body reacts to certain foods and physical activity.

Here are a few indicators that you may be an endomorph:

Inclination to acquire weight quickly, particularly around the belly.

Inability to lose weight even with conventional diet and activity plans.

Feeling that you are not as physically strong as your classmates.

Body type is mostly determined by genetics, but environmental variables like nutrition and lifestyle also have a big influence. Because of this, determining your body type also entails comprehending how these elements have shaped the composition and structure of your body throughout time.

Take into account these measures in order to determine your body type accurately:

Self-Analysis: Examine your physical attributes, such as muscular tone, body form, and fat distribution.

Keep an Eye on Your Metabolic Reactions: Keep an eye on how your body reacts to various diets and exercise regimens.

Professional Assessment: To have a more accurate picture, speak with a fitness or health specialist who is qualified to do body composition analyses and other evaluations.

Being an endomorph does not mean that you have to accept a life of low health or fitness. Rather, it involves being aware of and in harmony with your body's innate inclinations. Accepting your body type enables you to approach nutrition and exercise in a more individualized and successful way, producing better and longer-lasting benefits.

Characteristics of an Endomorph

Generally speaking, endomorphs have rounder, fuller figures. Physique fat is more common in this kind of physique and is often found in the belly, hips, and thighs. Compared to other body types, endomorphs often have less defined muscles, and they may have difficulty losing weight and keeping it off.

Important physical characteristics consist of:

Supple, rounded body form.

Broader waist and more substantial bone structure.

Propensity to readily accumulate fat.

Endomorphs are more likely to acquire weight due in large part to their metabolism. Endomorphs often burn calories more slowly than ectomorphs or mesomorphs because they have slower metabolic rates. Weight gain may result from this slowed metabolism, particularly if calorie intake is not strictly controlled.

Important metabolic characteristics consist of:

Decreased BMR, or basal metabolic rate.

Effective fat accumulation, often serving as a defense mechanism.

A challenge to burn off extra fat.

Endomorphs may also be subject to certain hormonal factors that impact their ability to control their weight and body composition. They often have higher sensitivity to the hormone insulin, which controls blood sugar levels, which increases their tendency to store fat, especially around the abdomen.

Additional hormone-related variables consist of:

Greater susceptibility to the weight-gaining effects of the stress hormone cortisol.

Possible abnormalities in the levels of the hormones leptin and ghrelin, which control hunger and fullness.

When it comes to nutrition and exercise, endomorphs often react differently than other body types. They could discover that steady-state aerobic activity programs and conventional low-calorie diets are less successful in helping them lose weight. Rather, a well-managed diet emphasizing macronutrient balance together with high-intensity interval training (HIIT) and strength training likely to be more successful.

Although having an endomorphic body type is normal and healthy, it's vital to be aware of the possible health issues that might arise if it's not properly controlled. Because of the propensity to retain visceral fat, these concerns may include an increased risk of insulin resistance, type 2 diabetes, and cardiovascular illnesses.

A comprehensive approach to exercise and wellness is crucial for endomorphs. This entails not just concentrating on weight loss but also taking into account variables such as stress reduction, quality of sleep, and mental health, all of which have a substantial influence on general health and body composition.

How Your Body Type Affects Your Metabolism Endomorph body types are inherently associated with certain metabolic inclinations. Endomorphs are mostly known for having slower metabolic rates. This implies that, in comparison to ectomorphs or mesomorphs, their bodies naturally burn less calories during rest and activity. Comprehending this essential element is crucial for customizing health and exercise regimens that work.

The pace at which your body burns calories or expends energy is known as its metabolic rate. Endomorphs often have lower basal metabolic rates (BMRs), or the amount of energy needed to maintain bodily functions when at rest. Weight control may become more difficult as a result of this slowed metabolism since the body prefers to retain extra calories rather than burn them.

Fat storage is an effective energy storage mechanism for endomorphs. While this feature is helpful in situations when food is scarce, it presents problems in contemporary settings where high-calorie items are easily accessible. Endomorphs are more inclined than other body types to retain extra calories as fat, especially in the abdomen, which increases their risk of obesity and associated health problems.

Hormones have a major influence on metabolic regulation, and endomorphs are more affected than other body types. For example, endomorphs may be more sensitive to insulin, which may result in more fat accumulation after meals high in carbohydrates. Hormones linked to stress, such as cortisol, may also affect how fat is stored.

Because of their slower metabolism and inclination to store fat, endomorphs often have more difficulty losing weight. Conventional diets that ignore these metabolic quirks may be less beneficial and, in some situations, even worsen the metabolic slowdown.

Dietary and exercise regimens may be more effectively tailored for endomorph body types by taking into account their metabolic preferences. In addition to reducing caloric intake, diets should target hormone balance and metabolic rate enhancement. Exercise regimens that include both cardio and strength training may be more successful in increasing metabolism and encouraging endomorphic fat reduction.

Endomorphs must embrace a well-rounded strategy that include dietary adjustments, physical activity, and lifestyle modifications. By using a comprehensive approach, it may be possible to manage the particular metabolic issues, encourage long-term weight reduction, and enhance general health.

3. THE SCIENCE BEHIND METABOLIC CONFUSION

Metabolic Rate and Adaptation

The pace at which the body uses energy or burns calories is referred to as its metabolic rate. It is essential for maintaining a healthy weight and general wellbeing. The metabolic rate is made up of two main parts:

Basal Metabolic Rate (BMR): The energy used up while the body is at rest. It makes up the bulk of a person's daily energy expenditure and is impacted by a number of variables, including body composition, age, gender, and heredity.

Calories burnt above and beyond resting levels during physical activity and everyday motions are included in the term "active metabolic rate."

An important factor in controlling weight is metabolism. A greater metabolic rate may help with weight reduction and prevent weight gain since it increases the amount of calories burned by the body both at rest and during activity. On the other hand, a decreased metabolic rate may facilitate weight gain and make weight reduction more difficult.

The term "metabolic adaptation," which is also used to describe adaptive thermogenesis, describes the body's capacity to modify its metabolic rate in response to variations in energy expenditure and calorie intake. This is an energy-saving survival strategy that the body uses when there is calorie restriction or heightened physical strain.

The body lowers its metabolic rate to preserve energy in response to prolonged, substantial calorie restriction. Although advantageous from an evolutionary standpoint, this adaptation may provide difficulties for long-term weight reduction and maintenance.

There might be a noticeable increase in metabolic adaptability in those with an endomorph body type. Endomorphs' slower metabolisms by nature make them more vulnerable to further metabolic slowdowns when calorie intake is continuously low, which makes long-term weight loss even more difficult.

The idea of Metabolic Confusion is to mitigate the consequences of metabolic adaptation. The diet seeks to avoid the metabolic slowing linked to conventional, continuous calorie-restricted diets by interspersing days of greater and lower calorie consumption.

The reasoning for this is that by maintaining uncertainty, the body's metabolic rate does not decrease and instead stays elevated. This may promote weight reduction and keep it from plateauing.

People who use Metabolic Confusion may benefit in a number of ways, such as:

Preventing Metabolic Slowdown: Keeping your metabolic rate higher may be achieved by adjusting your calorie intake on a regular basis.

Enhanced Fat Burning: The body may burn stored fat for energy more effectively if it has a more active metabolism.

Better Weight Loss Outcomes: People may find it simpler to keep losing weight over time if they prevent the adaption that stops weight loss.

Hormonal Factors Affecting Weight Loss

The body uses hormones as chemical messengers to control a number of physiological functions, including as hunger, metabolism, and fat storage. The way the body uses energy, breaks down food, and stores fat is all influenced by the balance of these hormones, and these functions are vital to controlling weight.

Numerous hormones have a major impact on weight growth and loss:

Insulin: The pancreas secretes insulin, a hormone that controls blood sugar levels. It influences fat metabolism and makes it easier for glucose to be stored as fat. Weight reduction might be more difficult if an overweight person has insulin resistance, which is a frequent problem.

Leptin: Also referred to as the satiety hormone, leptin is generated by fat cells and inhibits hunger, which aids in the regulation of energy balance. Overeating and weight gain may result from leptin resistance.

Often referred to as the "hunger hormone," ghrelin is mostly secreted in the stomach and instructs the brain to increase appetite. Elevated ghrelin levels may cause an increase in food consumption.

Cortisol: This hormone associated with stress has an impact on hunger and fat accumulation. Weight gain, particularly around the waist, may be attributed to elevated cortisol levels and chronic stress.

Hormone imbalances, both in this and other tissues, may have a major effect on attempts to control weight. For example, reduced leptin sensitivity combined with high insulin and cortisol levels may cause cravings, increased appetite, and fat accumulation, all of which impede weight reduction.

Through food diversity, the Metabolic Confusion diet may indirectly affect hormonal homeostasis. This diet may help regulate hormones like insulin and leptin by alternating between days with higher and lower calories, which may improve sensitivity and decrease resistance.

Enhanced Insulin Sensitivity: Altering calorie intake on a regular basis may help avoid persistently elevated insulin levels, which lowers the chance of developing insulin resistance.

Leptin and Ghrelin Balance: A varied diet may have a good effect on the levels of leptin and ghrelin, which may lessen excessive hunger and help regulate appetite.

Diminished Cortisol Effect: By reducing the stress reaction and providing enough calories, a well-balanced diet may help bring down cortisol levels.

The Metabolic Confusion diet is a potential method for endomorphs, who may be more susceptible to hormone abnormalities impacting weight. It offers a diverse and well-balanced food pattern that may assist with some of the particular hormonal issues that this body type faces.

The Mechanism of Metabolic Confusion
Caloric fluctuation is the central concept of Metabolic Confusion. This method alternates between times when calorie intake is greater and lower, in contrast to standard diets that maintain a steady calorie intake. Depending on the requirements and objectives of each person, this variation may happen on a daily, weekly, or other scheduled cycle basis.

Preventing metabolic adaptation, a condition in which the body modifies its metabolic rate to meet calorie intake and often results in a weight loss plateau, is one of the main goals of Metabolic Confusion. The body cannot completely adjust when calorie intake is continuously fluctuating, which may maintain a higher and more active metabolic rate.

Metabolic Confusion seeks to activate the metabolism in many ways by varying the calorie levels:

The body gets more energy than normal during high-calorie phases, which may momentarily raise the metabolic rate. Additionally, this may help with muscle development and recuperation, particularly when paired with weight exercise.

The body is urged to use fat reserves as energy during low-calorie phases, which results in weight reduction. This impact of burning fat can be strengthened by the contrast with high-calorie times.

The body's hormonal reactions to food may also be influenced by metabolic confusion:

Insulin Sensitivity: Because the body cycles between periods of greater and lower carbohydrate consumption, varying the amount of carbohydrates consumed may help enhance insulin sensitivity.

Changes in calorie intake may have an impact on the levels of the hunger-related hormones leptin and ghrelin, which might help manage appetite.

Metabolic confusion has psychological advantages in addition to physiological ones. Diets with greater flexibility and diversity tend to be less restrictive and more sustainable than conventional diets, which increases adherence and pleasure.

Metabolic confusion may be especially helpful for endomorphs, who often battle with a slower metabolism and a higher predisposition for fat accumulation. The varied calorie intake of the diet is in line with the requirement to boost fat burning and rev up a sluggish metabolism.

In order to successfully use Metabolic Confusion, it is important that:

Recognize Your Unique Calorie Requirements: Adjust calories based on your objectives, activity level, and metabolic rate.

Preserve Nutritional Balance: Pay attention to the quality of macronutrients and make sure that both high- and low-calorie days are nutritionally balanced.

Monitor and Modify: Evaluate progress on a regular basis and make necessary modifications in light of feedback and outcomes.

4. DEVELOPING A CUSTOMIZED MEAL PLAN

Creating the Perfect Plate

Recognizing your own dietary requirements is the first step towards creating your dream meal. This entails taking into account variables like your exercise level, food preferences, basal metabolic rate, and any particular health concerns. A varied range of nutrients, such as proteins, carbs, fats, vitamins, and minerals, should be included in a balanced diet.

A well-planned plate should include an equal distribution of the three main macronutrients:

Proteins: An important component of any diet, proteins aid in the formation and repair of muscles. Pick lean foods such as fish, poultry, tofu, lentils, and low-fat dairy.

Your body uses carbohydrates as its main energy source. Choose complex carbs for long-lasting energy and fiber, such as those found in whole grains, fruits, and vegetables.

Healthy fats are essential for the synthesis of hormones and the absorption of nutrients. Incorporate sources such as nuts, seeds, avocados, and olive oil, but in moderation.

Your plate will have varying amounts of calories in accordance with the Metabolic Confusion approach:

On days when you need to consume extra calories, you may load your plate with additional healthy fats and carbs. Additionally, it is a wonderful time to include higher-calorie, nutrient-dense foods in your diet.

On low-calorie days, reduce your intake of carbohydrates and fats and instead concentrate on meals high in fiber and protein that will keep you fuller for longer.

The key to controlling calorie consumption is portion management. When determining portion sizes, use visual cues: a serving of protein should be the size of your palm, a portion of carbs should be the size of your closed fist, and a serving of fats should not exceed a tiny handful.

Not only does variety guarantee a broad range of nutrients in meals, it also keeps them interesting. To guarantee complete nutrition, rotate various protein sources, fruits, vegetables, and whole grains throughout your meal plan.

Any dietary requirements or preferences you may have, such as vegetarian, vegan, gluten-free, or lactose-intolerant alternatives, should also be taken into account when designing your perfect plate. Making a food plan that fits your lifestyle and is sustainable, pleasurable, and pleasant is the aim.

Plan nutritious snacks in addition to your main meals to help you control your appetite and stay energized all day. Think of nutrient-dense snacks like fruits, almonds, yogurt, or whole-grain crackers that are in line with your daily calorie objectives.

Observe how your body reacts to various meals and serving sizes. As you go, you may need to make adjustments based on things like hunger, energy levels, and general contentment.

Balancing Macronutrients

Every macronutrient has a distinct function that is vital to the body:

Proteins: The building blocks of muscle, skin, enzymes, and hormones, proteins are essential for the development and repair of tissues.

The body uses carbohydrates as its main energy source; they are especially crucial for mental and physical activities.

Fats: Essential for several processes, such as the synthesis of hormones, the absorption of nutrients, and the provision of a concentrated energy source.

Based on individual characteristics including body type, metabolic rate, exercise level, and personal health objectives, the proper balance of these macronutrients might change. For the distribution of macronutrients, a common rule of thumb may be:

25–35% of total calories come from protein.

40–50% of total calories come from carbohydrates, with complex carbs accounting for the majority of energy.

20–35% of calories come from fats, mostly unsaturated fats.

A Metabolic Confusion diet will cause these ratios to change:

On days when you need more calories, increase the amount of healthy fats and carbs you eat while keeping your protein consumption same.

On days when you're on a low-calorie diet, try to keep your protein consumption greater to help with satiety and muscle maintenance and lower your intake of fats and carbs.

The quality of macronutrients is equally as important as their quantity:

Select Lean Proteins: Go for foods like eggs, salmon, tofu, lentils, and chicken breast.

Choose Complex Carbohydrates: Include fruits, vegetables, whole grains, and legumes.

Choose Good Fats: Give special attention to foods like avocados, almonds, seeds, and olive oil.

It is important to keep track of how your body reacts to various macronutrient balances:

Pay Attention to Your Body: Keep an eye on your energy levels, hunger signals, and post-meal mood after consuming various kinds of food.

As necessary, adjust: Adjust the macronutrient ratios to see what suits you best, taking into account your findings and observations.

Your workout regimen may also alter your demands for macronutrients:

On Workout Days: Especially during your workouts, you could need additional carbs for energy.

During days of rest, you may consume a higher proportion of proteins and fats since your body may need less energy.

To assist monitor and modify your consumption of macronutrients, think about using resources like as meal diaries, apps, or speaking with a nutritionist. This may provide you important information about your eating habits and assist you in making wise changes.

7-Day Sample Meal Plans for Endomorphs

Day 1: High-Calorie Day

- Breakfast: Scrambled eggs with spinach, whole grain toast, and avocado.
- Lunch: Grilled chicken breast with quinoa salad and mixed vegetables.
- Snack: Greek yogurt with mixed berries and a handful of almonds.
- Dinner: Baked salmon with sweet potato and steamed broccoli.
- Dessert: Dark chocolate square and a small serving of mixed fruit.

Day 2: Low-Calorie Day

- Breakfast: Oatmeal with sliced banana and a sprinkle of cinnamon.
- Lunch: Lentil soup with a side salad (leafy greens and cherry tomatoes).
- Snack: Carrot sticks with hummus.
- Dinner: Stir-fried tofu with mixed bell peppers and brown rice.
- Evening Snack: Cottage cheese with a few pineapple chunks.

Day 3: High-Calorie Day

- Breakfast: Whole grain pancakes topped with fresh strawberries and a drizzle of honey.
- Lunch: Turkey and cheese sandwich on whole grain bread with lettuce and tomato, and a side of sweet potato fries.
- Snack: Apple slices with peanut butter.
- Dinner: Beef stir-fry with brown rice and mixed vegetables.
- Dessert: Small bowl of fruit salad.

Day 4: Low-Calorie Day

- Breakfast: Green smoothie (spinach, kale, green apple, and a scoop of protein powder).
- Lunch: Grilled chicken salad with mixed greens, cucumber, and a vinaigrette dressing.
- Snack: A hard-boiled egg.
- Dinner: Grilled shrimp with zucchini noodles and marinara sauce.
- Evening Snack: A small handful of mixed nuts.

Day 5: High-Calorie Day

- Breakfast: Avocado toast on whole grain bread with poached eggs.
- Lunch: Tuna salad wrap with whole grain tortilla and a side of mixed fruit.
- Snack: Protein shake with a banana.
- Dinner: Pork chop with roasted Brussels sprouts and mashed potatoes.
- Dessert: A scoop of gelato or sorbet.

Day 6: Low-Calorie Day

- Breakfast: Greek yogurt with a sprinkle of granola and fresh blueberries.
- Lunch: Vegetable stir-fry with tofu and a small serving of brown rice.
- Snack: Sliced cucumber with a sprinkle of chili and lime.
- Dinner: Baked cod with a side of asparagus and quinoa.
- Evening Snack: A piece of dark chocolate.

Day 7: High-Calorie Day

- Breakfast: Banana and walnut oatmeal with a splash of almond milk.

- Lunch: Chicken Caesar salad with croutons and parmesan cheese.

- Snack: Mixed nuts and dried fruit.

- Dinner: Lasagna with a side of garlic bread and a green salad.

- Dessert: Baked apple with cinnamon and a dollop of whipped cream.

5. EXERCISE TECHNIQUES FOR METABOLIC CONFUSION

Strength and cardio exercise combined has various advantages for those following the Metabolic Confusion diet:

Enhanced Fat Loss: Strength training improves muscle, which raises metabolic rate, and cardio helps burn calories and fat.

Enhanced muscular Tone: Lean muscular mass is developed via strength training, which enhances overall body composition.

Enhanced Metabolic Flexibility: By assisting the body in smoothly transitioning between various energy sources, this combination strategy improves metabolic flexibility.

Cardio and strength training should be balanced in a well-designed exercise program:

Frequency: Depending on your objectives and level of fitness, aim for three to five days of mixed exercise each week.

Intensity: Change up how hard you work out. Incorporate both lower-repetition, heavier lifting for strength and high-intensity interval training (HIIT) for cardio.

Duration: Training sessions may last anywhere from 30 to 60 minutes, with equal emphasis placed on strength and aerobic training.

It takes cardiovascular activity to burn calories and strengthen the heart:

HIIT (sprint intervals, circuit training) and steady-state cardio (cycling, running) are examples of different types of cardio.

Timing: To optimize fat burning and muscle repair, think about doing cardio after strength training or on different days.

Customization: Pick aerobic activities that you like, that match your fitness level, and that are good for your joints.

Strength exercise is crucial for increasing metabolism and gaining muscle:

When choosing exercises, pay attention to complex motions that target many muscular groups, such as bench presses, deadlifts, and squats.

Progressive Overload: To keep pushing your muscles, gradually increase the weight, repetitions, or sets over time.

Recovery: To promote muscular development and recovery, make sure you get enough sleep in between strength training sessions.

Complement your diet for Metabolic Confusion with exercise:

High-Calorie Days: Make the most of the additional energy by concentrating on longer, more intense strength training sessions.

Exercise lightly or shorter, or concentrate more on cardio, on low-calorie days.

Utilize metrics like as increased strength, increased endurance, and altered body composition to monitor your progress. Adapt your workout regimen as necessary to your new diet and fitness objectives.

In any fitness endeavor, consistency is essential. Remember that decreasing weight and gaining muscle takes time, so be patient with your progress.

High-Intensity Interval Training (HIIT)
Short bursts of intensive exercise are interspersed with rest or lower-intensity activity during high-intensity interval training (HIIT). This kind of exercise is well-known for raising metabolic rate, enhancing fat burning, and strengthening cardiovascular health.

Enhanced Fat Burning: By causing a metabolic disruption that burns calories long after a workout (the after burn effect), HIIT speeds up the loss of fat.

Better Cardiovascular Health: By fortifying the heart and lungs, it raises cardiovascular fitness levels all around.

Time Efficiency: While providing substantial health advantages, high-intensity interval training (HIIT) sessions may be shorter than regular cardio exercises.

Elevated Metabolic Rate: The high intensity of high-intensity interval training (HIIT) may raise your body's metabolic rate for hours after you work out.

An HIIT workout may be organized as follows and can run anywhere from 15 to 30 minutes on average:

Warm-up: To get the body ready, start with five to ten minutes of gentle aerobic activity.

High-Intensity Intervals: Engage in high-intensity activities such as burpees, jumping jacks, and running for brief intervals of 30 to 60 seconds.

Recovery Intervals: After every high-intensity burst, take a short break or engage in a low-intensity activity, such as walking or moderate jogging, for a duration that is typically twice or equal to the high-intensity intervals.

Repeat: Throughout the whole exercise, switch between high-intensity and rest periods.

Cool Down: To help with recuperation, stretch throughout the last five to ten minutes of your workout.

Because HIIT has the ability to dramatically increase metabolic rate and improve fat burning two essential components in controlling an endomorph's sluggish metabolism it may be very helpful for endomorphs.

Days with a lot of calories consumed: HIIT may be more beneficial since your body can exert itself to a greater extent.

On days when you're cutting calories, think about doing shorter or milder HIIT workouts or switching up your workout routine to avoid overtraining.

Although HIIT works, it is also really hard. It's critical to:

Start Modestly: If you're not familiar with HIIT, start with shorter workouts and progressively up the ante.

Pay Attention to Your Body: Observe your body's reaction and adjust the workouts accordingly.

Rest and Recover: To avoid overtraining and injury, make sure you get enough rest in between HIIT workouts.

Track gains in strength, endurance, and general fitness in addition to weight reduction. Frequent evaluations might assist in adjusting the frequency and intensity of HIIT exercises to your changing fitness requirements.

Adaptive Workout Programs

Exercise programs that are adaptive are dynamic and adaptable, meant to change with the body as it needs them to. This strategy is essential for those on the Metabolic Confusion diet because it matches the kind and intensity of exercise to the diet's varying calorie intake.

Consistent with Dietary Phases: Exercises may be designed to balance days with high and low caloric intake, guaranteeing maximum energy use and recuperation.

Personalization: By adapting to each person's fitness level, preferences, and objectives, adaptive routines may boost motivation and efficiency.

Prevents Plateaus: By continuously pushing the body and encouraging advancement, rotating training regimens helps avoid fitness plateaus.

When creating adaptive workout programs, a number of elements must be taken into account:

Exercise Variety: Include HIIT, weight training, cardio, and flexibility exercises. This diversity keeps exercises engaging while simultaneously promoting general health.

Workout Intensity: Modify the level of intensity to correspond with the body's energy capacity. Plan harder exercises on days when your energy intake is high and lighter activities on days when your energy intake is low.

Progressive Overload: To keep your body challenged, progressively raise the ante on training intensity, duration, or complexity.

Here's a sample week that adapts to the Metabolic Confusion diet:

Monday (High-Calorie Day): Intense strength training focusing on major muscle groups.

Tuesday (Low-Calorie Day): Light cardio such as walking or a gentle cycling session.

Wednesday (High-Calorie Day): HIIT session or a more intense cardio workout.

Thursday (Low-Calorie Day): Yoga or Pilates for flexibility and core strength.

Friday (High-Calorie Day): Strength training with a focus on different muscle groups from Monday.

Saturday (Low-Calorie Day): Active recovery with activities like light swimming or a leisurely walk.

Sunday: Rest day or light stretching to aid recovery.

Keep an eye on your responses: Observe how your body feels both during and after exercise. Weariness, persistent pain, or a lack of improvement might be signs that something needs to change.

Be Adaptable: Be ready to adjust your regimen in response to changes in your energy level, your lifestyle, or any arising physical difficulties.

Exercises alone are not as vital as rest and recovery:

Schedule Rest Days: To give the body time to heal, try to schedule at least one complete rest day per week.

Incorporate Active Recovery: On rest days, low-intensity exercises like walking or light stretching may help with recovery.

Achieving long-term success with an adaptive workout regimen requires consistency. Recall that patience is necessary and that progress could be slow.

6. HOW AND WHEN TO EAT

Intermittent Fasting for Endomorphs

Cycling between eating and fasting phases is known as intermittent fasting. When it comes to eating, IF focuses more on when than what to consume, unlike standard diets. Two popular IF techniques are the 16/8 approach, which involves fasting for 16 hours and eating within an 8-hour window, and the 5:2 method, which involves five days of regular eating followed by two days of calorie restriction.

Endomorphs are better at storing energy as fat and often have slower metabolisms. IF may work well for endomorphs since it can:

Improve Metabolic Flexibility: It makes the body more adept at alternating between burning fat and carbohydrates for energy.

Boost Insulin Sensitivity: Frequent fasting intervals may help control blood sugar levels and enhance the body's reaction to insulin.

Boost Fat Loss: If you combine intermittent fasting (IF) with the Metabolic Confusion diet, the length of time your body spends fasting may help you burn more fat.

Select the Appropriate Approach: Begin with a less restricted IF strategy, such the 16/8 technique, then modify according to your experience.

Comply with Metabolic Distortion: To optimize fat burning on your low-calorie days, schedule fasting times.

Eat Balanced Meals: Concentrate on nutrient-dense meals that meet your calorie and macronutrient targets throughout your eating windows.

Track Energy Levels: Keep an eye on your body's reactions to fasting, particularly how it affects your appetite and energy levels.

Modify Depending on Activity: To guarantee enough energy and recuperation after demanding exercises, think about cutting short the fasting times.

Keep Yourself Hydrated: Throughout the day, particularly while fasting, sip plenty of water.

Exercise Timing: To optimize fat burning, some people find it helpful to work out close to the conclusion of their fast. But depending on personal tastes and energy levels, this may change.

Post-Workout Nutrition: Make sure the food you have after working out is balanced, nutrient-dense, and meets your daily calorie target.

Handling Hunger: At first, during fasting times, you may feel hungrier. You may control your appetite by consuming black coffee, herbal teas, or water.

A Look at Social and Lifestyle Factors Schedule your fasting times to avoid interfering with family dinners or social gatherings.

Monitor Your Development: To track changes in your weight, energy levels, body composition, and general well-being, keep a diary.

Be Patient and Adaptable: Adaptation takes time, so make any necessary adjustments to your fasting routine.

Optimizing Meal Timing
Your metabolism, energy levels, and the overall efficacy of your diet may all be greatly impacted by the time of your meals. You may improve nutrition

absorption, control appetite, and promote metabolic health by coordinating your meal schedule with your body's normal functions and daily activity levels.

Breakfast: Eating a healthy meal first thing in the morning helps boost your metabolism and provide you energy throughout the day. A breakfast high in protein may assist endomorphs control their blood sugar levels.

Lunch: Eating a healthy, balanced meal can help you stay energetic all afternoon. A combination of complex carbs, healthy fats, and proteins should be included.

Dinner: Since your metabolism slows down near the end of the day, your evening meal should be lighter. Avoid consuming too many carbs and instead concentrate on veggies and lean meats.

Pre-Workout Meals: For energy, if you work out, think about having a modest, high-carb snack or meal one to two hours beforehand.

Post-Workout Meals: To promote muscle repair and restock glycogen reserves, eat a post-workout meal high in proteins and carbs.

Regular Meals: Eating at regular times may assist control your body's metabolic reactions and hunger signals. Try to eat three major meals a day, and you may choose to include or exclude snacks based on your own requirements and tastes.

Snacking: Select foods high in nutrients, such as fruits, almonds, or yogurt, if you decide to snack. The timing of snacks may help control hunger and provide energy in between meals.

Your metabolism is influenced by your circadian rhythm, which is your body's internal clock. Eating in a way that is consistent with your circadian cycle may improve metabolic and digestive efficiency. Keep your calorie intake mostly throughout the day and avoid eating too much at night.

Spread out your calories more evenly across the day on high-calorie days to accommodate your increased energy requirements. If you're on a low-calorie diet, think about cutting down on the amount of your meals or skipping the snack.

Monitor Your Reactions: Take note of how eating at various times affects your digestion, energy levels, and general health.

Be Adaptable: Be flexible with meal timings to accommodate your daily routine, hunger signals, and energy needs.

Meal Planning: Arrange your meals ahead of time to make sure they complement your daily schedule and nutritional objectives.

Consistency: To aid in regulating your body's internal clock, try eating at around the same times every day.

Eating mindfully involves paying attention to your body's cues about hunger and fullness. Mindful eating may help with digestion and stop overindulging.

Handling Cravings and Hunger

Firstly, it's critical to differentiate between cravings a strong yearning for certain foods that are often motivated by emotional factors and hunger, which is the body's need for food. To effectively handle each, it is essential to understand their differences.

Physical hunger: gradual, satiable with a variety of meals, disappears when sated.

Emotional Cravings: Severe, non-physically driven desires for certain meals.

Effectively controlling hunger entails:

Eating Frequently: Being too hungry might result from missing meals. To keep blood sugar levels stable, eat at regular intervals.

Including Fiber and Protein: These are necessary nutrients for feeling full. Every meal and snack should include a source of fiber and protein.

Maintaining Hydration: Occasionally, hunger and thirst are confused. Make sure you have plenty water to drink throughout the day.

Consciously Consuming Food: Observe the signals your body sends whether it is hungry or full. Eating should be done quietly and slowly.

Here are some ways to control cravings:

Identifying Triggers: Recognize the things that make you need certain foods, such as stress, boredom, emotional anguish, etc., and come up with other strategies to deal with these emotions.

Wholesome alternatives Find satisfying substitutes that will not break your diet. For instance, choose fresh fruit over sugary snacks or dark chocolate over milk chocolate.

Portion Control: Give in to your cravings, but only in little amounts. Preparing sweets in advance may help prevent overindulgence.

Regular Meal Times: Eating at regular intervals might help control appetite and lessen cravings.

Balanced Meals: To keep you satiated for longer, make sure each meal contains a proper ratio of fats, carbs, and proteins.

Aligning with Metabolic Confusion: To avoid hunger on low-calorie days, concentrate on eating a lot of low-calorie items like vegetables and lean proteins.

Emotional Eating: Recognize your emotional eating habits and look for healthy coping mechanisms, such as hobbies, exercise, or meditation.

Positive Reinforcement: Give yourself something other than food as a reward for making healthy decisions. Some ideas include a soothing bath, a new book, or time spent doing a favorite activity.

Lifestyle Adjustments: Make sure you get enough sleep, exercise often, and practice stress reduction.

Education: Get to know nutrition and the effects that various foods have on your body and emotions.

Professional Advice: See a nutritionist or counselor if your hunger and cravings are severe or hard to control.

Support Groups: Connecting with others in similar situations may provide guidance and words of encouragement.

7. FOODS YOU SHOULD LOVE AND AVOID

Endomorph-Friendly Foods

Endomorphs tend to accumulate fat more readily and have slower metabolisms. As a result, the majority of the meals in their diet should be ones that may increase metabolism, prolong satiety, and give long-lasting energy. It's important to prioritize low-calorie, high-nutrient meals and to watch portion sizes.

For endomorphs, proteins are necessary because they promote muscular growth, satiety, and an increased metabolic rate.

Lean Meats: Turkey, lean beef or pig chops, and chicken breast.

Fish: Omega-3 fatty acid-rich fatty fish such as mackerel, salmon, and tuna.

Plant-based proteins include tempeh, tofu, beans, and lentils.

Long-lasting energy is provided by complex carbs, which don't cause blood sugar levels to rise.

Whole Grains: whole grain bread, barley, quinoa, and brown rice.

Broccoli, Brussels sprouts, bell peppers, and leafy greens are examples of fibrous vegetables.

Fruits with low Glycemic Index: oranges, pears, apples, and berries.

Good fats are essential for the synthesis of hormones and general well-being.

Nuts and Seeds: Chia seeds, flaxseeds, walnuts, and almonds.

One excellent source of monounsaturated fats is avocados.

Oils: In moderation, use coconut oil, olive oil, and other plant-based oils.

Hydration is essential.

The greatest option for keeping hydrated is water.

Herbal teas: For individuals who like something more flavored than water, these might be an excellent substitute.

Fiber helps in digestion, maintaining gut health, and keeping you full longer.

Vegetables: Particularly green, leafy vegetables.

Whole Grains: As mentioned above, along with whole grain pasta and cereals.

Legumes: Such as beans, lentils, and chickpeas.

Foods with a low to moderate glycemic index are preferred as they cause a slower, more gradual increase in blood sugar levels.

Whole Fruits: Rather than fruit juices.

Dairy: Low-fat or non-fat options like Greek yogurt or cottage cheese.

Healthy snacking is important to manage hunger and provide energy throughout the day.

Vegetable Sticks: With hummus or Greek yogurt dip.

Fruit: Paired with a handful of nuts for protein.

Protein Smoothies: Using plant-based protein powder, leafy greens, and a small amount of fruit.

Even if endomorph-friendly meals are the major emphasis, it's crucial to have a balanced diet. Every food group has significance, and it is not advised to completely exclude any group unless it is absolutely required by medicine.

Finally, it's critical to customize your diet depending on your unique interests, lifestyle, and reaction to various meals. Even within the same body type, what works for one individual could not work for another.

Foods to Reduce or Stop Eating
Processed Sugars: Candy, baked goods, and sugary drinks are examples of foods rich in processed sugars that may cause blood sugar and insulin levels to surge, which encourages the accumulation of fat.

Artificial Sweeteners: Despite having little calories, artificial sweeteners may cause appetite management issues and elicit cravings for sweet foods.

White bread and pasta may cause sharp rises in blood sugar since they don't have the same amount of fiber as their whole grain equivalents.

Processed Snacks: Chips, crackers, and other processed snacks are often high in harmful fats and refined carbohydrates.

Trans Fats: Often included in baked products, fried meals, and processed snack items, trans fats raise the risk of inflammation and heart disease.

Saturated Fats: Although certain saturated fats are not bad for you, you should only eat them occasionally. Limit your use of full-fat dairy products and high-fat meat cuts.

Empty Calories: Alcohol has little nutritional benefits and contains calories that might make you gain weight.

Alcohol Use: Consuming alcohol may increase hunger and lower inhibitions about food, which might result in overindulging.

Heavy in Calories: These foods often lack important nutrients but are heavy in calories, bad fats, and salt.

Preservatives and additives: When ingested in excess, additives and preservatives found in many processed foods may be hazardous to one's health.

Energy drinks and sodas: These sugar-laden drinks may add a lot of calories to your diet without offering any nutritious value or satisfaction.

Fruit Juices: Even pure fruit juices may have low fiber content and high sugar content.

Excess Sodium: Consuming a lot of sodium, which is often included in salty foods, may cause high blood pressure and water retention.

Foods for Snacks: Salty snacks such as chips and pretzels may be overindulgent and addicting.

Moderation: It could be impractical and unsustainable to completely give up on certain meals. Rather, emphasize restraint and deliberate overindulgence.

Wholesome alternatives Seek for better options to sate hunger. For example, go for air-popped popcorn instead of chips or dark chocolate instead of light chocolate.

Reading Nutrition Labels: Develop your ability to read nutrition labels to spot added salt, bad fats, and hidden sugars.

Preventing Deprivation: Strict diets may cause people to feel as if they are depriving themselves, which may lead to binge eating. It's crucial to strike a balance between regular pleasures and a balanced diet.

Eating with awareness: Become aware of your eating patterns and develop the ability to discriminate between emotional and physical urges.

8. SUPPLEMENTS

Vitamins and Minerals for Endomorphs

Endomorphs often have unique difficulties with energy levels, fat storage, and metabolism. Sufficient consumption of certain vitamins and minerals may aid in resolving these problems, promoting general well-being, and augmenting the efficiency of the Metabolic Confusion diet.

Vitamin D: Essential for strong bones and a healthy immune system. It could possibly be involved in mood regulation and the avoidance of mood swings.

B vitamins are a class of vitamins that are essential for the metabolism of energy. For endomorphs in particular, B12 is crucial because it facilitates the transformation of food into energy.

Vitamin C serves as an antioxidant and enhances immune system performance. Additionally, it's critical for the manufacture of collagen, which is essential for healthy skin and joints.

Magnesium: Involved in more than 300 enzymatic processes, including muscle and energy metabolism, throughout the body.

Calcium: Necessary for healthy bones and muscles. Endomorphs need to consume enough calcium, particularly if they are strength training.

Iron: Vital for general health and energy levels. Fatigue brought on by an iron shortage might impair general vigor and exercise performance.

Omega-3 Fatty Acids: These vital fats may help lower inflammation and are crucial for heart health.

Fiber: Although it isn't a vitamin or mineral, fiber is vital for gastrointestinal health and may help control weight by increasing fullness.

Prior to beginning a supplement program, make sure you:

Speak with a Medical Professional: Make sure the supplements you are thinking about are suitable for your particular requirements.

Supplement Quality: Select reliable, high-quality products to guarantee effectiveness and safety.

Dosage and Timing: Take into account the timing of supplements, especially in relation to meals and activity, and adhere to suggested amounts.

Vitamins and minerals are best obtained via natural dietary sources, while supplements have their uses as well. To meet the majority of your nutritional requirements, concentrate on eating a balanced diet full of fruits, vegetables, whole grains, lean meats, and healthy fats.

Keep an eye on how supplements affect your body's reaction. It's crucial to monitor and make any required adjustments to supplements since some of them may have adverse effects or interfere with drugs.

Herbal Supplements

Supplements containing herbs may provide a natural means of supporting different body processes. They may help weight reduction, boost energy levels, improve metabolism, and have positive effects on general health. But it's crucial to approach using herbal supplements sensibly and intelligently.

Green tea extract is well-known for increasing metabolism and burning fat. Caffeine and catechins found in green tea may help in weight reduction.

Ginseng: This plant is said to increase vitality and assist control blood sugar, which is especially advantageous for endomorphs.

Curcumin, a substance with anti-inflammatory and antioxidant qualities found in turmeric, may benefit general health.

Cinnamon: May lessen the chance of insulin surges, which may result in the accumulation of fat by regulating blood sugar levels.

Ginger: Well-known for its anti-inflammatory and digestive properties, ginger may help regulate hunger.

When thinking about using herbal supplements, it's important to:

Do your homework and learn about the advantages and possible drawbacks of any herbal product.

Quality and Purity: To guarantee efficacy and purity, choose premium goods from reliable vendors.

Consultation: Talk to your doctor about this, particularly if you take any other drugs or have pre-existing medical issues.

Complementary Strategy: Use herbal supplements in addition to a well-balanced diet, not in substitute of sensible eating practices.

Timing and Dosage: For optimal efficacy, adhere to suggested doses and think about the ideal moment to take the supplement.

Interactions with Prescription Drugs: The efficacy of some herbal supplements may be altered when used with prescription drugs.

Side Effects: If you have any negative reactions, stop using the product right away.

See How Your Body Reacts: Keep an eye on how your body reacts to herbal supplements and modify your dosage as needed.

Frequent Evaluations: Review the need of continuing supplementing on a regular basis, as certain supplements could be more advantageous in the near run.

Research-Based Decisions: Make dietary supplement selections based on facts, not fashion.

Long-Term Health Focus: Give up on short-term solutions in favor of long-term health and metabolic equilibrium.

9. OVERCOMING OBSTACLES AND PLATEAUS

Overcoming Weight Loss Plateaus

When you maintain your food and exercise regimen but stop losing weight, you may be experiencing a weight loss plateau. It's a typical phase of weight reduction and often an indication that your body has adjusted to your new routine.

Metabolic Adaptation: Your body needs less calories as you lose weight, which causes your metabolism to slow down.

Reduced Muscle Mass: If strength training isn't a part of your weight reduction plan, you may experience a decrease in muscle mass, which may slow down your metabolism.

Dietary Practices: Plateaus may be caused by either overestimating caloric expenditure or underestimating calorie intake.

Reevaluate Calorie Needs: Your calorie requirements drop as you shed pounds. Determine your calorie needs again using your present weight.

Boost Physical Activity: Extend the length of your physical activity, add additional exercises, or raise the intensity of your current routine.

Include Strength Training: Gaining muscle may help you overcome a plateau and raise your metabolic rate.

Change up Your training Routine: You may push your body in novel methods and rekindle weight loss by altering up your training regimen.

Adjust Your Diet: Consider again the foods and serving sizes you choose.

Modify Calorie Cycling: Modify the number of calories consumed on days that are high and low in calories.

Play around with the ratios of macronutrients: Adjust the ratios of fats, proteins, and carbs a little bit to see whether it affects weight reduction.

To make sure you're eating for bodily need rather than habit or emotion, pay attention to mindful eating.

Achievable and Realistic objectives: Establish attainable objectives for weight reduction. Recognize that weight loss is often nonlinear.

Patience: Recognize that reaching a plateau in your weight reduction efforts is common and will need perseverance and patience to get beyond.

Measure Body Composition: To get a more comprehensive view of your progress, use body measurements or body fat percentage to monitor changes.

Non-Scale Triumphs: Honor gains in energy, physical fitness, and clothing fit all of which may serve as markers of advancement even in the absence of a shift on the scale.

Professional Assistance: Consult a personal trainer, dietician, or healthcare professional for guidance if you continue to reach plateaus.

Support Groups: Talking with others who are going through similar things about your experiences and tactics might inspire you and give you fresh ideas.

Stress Reduction and Emotional Eating

Consuming food to satisfy emotional demands instead of physical hunger is known as emotional eating. This reaction may be brought on by stress, grief, boredom, or even pleasure, which can result in unhealthful eating habits that undermine nutritional objectives.

Self-Awareness: To see trends in your eating behaviors, keep a food journal. Keep track of your food intake, timing, and feelings.

Common Triggers: Emotions such as boredom, loneliness, stress, and other feelings might cause people to turn to food for solace.

Mindful Eating: Consider if you are eating out of emotion or hunger. Eating mindfully may assist in differentiating between the two.

Healthy Substitutes: Look for other coping mechanisms, including exercise, hobbies, or relaxation methods, to manage your emotions.

Emotional Support: Rather of using food as a consolation, discuss your emotions with friends, family, or specialists.

Effective stress management is essential as stress may trigger emotional eating.

Exercise: Getting regular exercise might help you feel happier and decrease stress.

Relaxation Techniques: Stress may be reduced by engaging in techniques like yoga, meditation, or deep breathing.

Sufficient Sleep: Make sure you receive enough good sleep, since insufficient sleep may lead to stress and change eating patterns.

Time management: Plan your days to make them less stressful. Set priorities for your work and make time for leisure and recuperation.

Frequent Meals: Eating on a regular basis may help control hunger and lessen the chance of emotional eating.

A well-balanced diet that emphasizes whole foods might help lower cravings and improve your mood.

Eat foods that are proven to alleviate stress, such as those that are rich in magnesium and omega-3 fatty acids.

Underlying Issues: Recognize that emotional eating is often a sign of more serious problems. Longer-lasting and more efficient solutions may result from addressing these underlying problems.

Modifications to Lifestyle: Include activities that enhance general well-being in your daily routine, such as socializing, engaging in hobbies and interests, and frequent physical exercise.

Staying Motivated and Consistent
The first choice to begin a diet and exercise program is driven by motivation, but long-term outcomes need persistence. Both are essential for breaking through plateaus and reaching long-term fitness and health objectives.

SMART Objectives: Establish objectives that are Time-bound, Relevant, Specific, Measurable, and Achievable.

Small, Gradual Objectives: Divide your primary objective into more achievable, smaller goals.

Social Support: Be in the company of encouraging friends, relatives, or a group of people who have similar aspirations.

Progress tracking: Use apps or a notebook to record your workouts, food, and progress toward your objectives.

Honor significant anniversaries: No matter how little, acknowledge and applaud each accomplishment. This may increase your drive.

Personal Motivation: Consider the reasons that are unique to you for wanting to become healthier and reduce weight. This 'why' has the potential to be an effective motivator.

Visual Cues: Place visible reminders of your objectives and motivations in areas you will often be exposed to.

Resilience: Recognize that obstacles are common. How you recover is what counts.

Learn from Mistakes: Make the most of failures to hone your strategy.

Positive Self-Talk: Switch out your negative ideas with empowering statements.

Mindfulness and Stress Reduction: Techniques like meditation may support stress reduction and the upkeep of an optimistic outlook.

Adapt to Changes: Be prepared to modify your workout and nutrition regimen as necessary. You can maintain consistency in the face of life's unpredictable events by being flexible.

Try new meals, recipes, and exercise routines without fear if you reach a plateau or lose interest.

Pleasurable Exercises: Select physical pursuits that you find enjoyable. If a habit is fun, you're more likely to continue with it.

Lifestyle Integration: Look for methods to include physical exercise into your everyday schedule, such as riding your bike to work or taking walks during breaks.

Educate Yourself: Continue to learn about exercise and nutrition. You may stay motivated and interested by continuing to study.

10. 21 DAY RECIPES AND MEAL PREP TIPS

21 Day Recipes

Day 1:

- Breakfast: Scrambled eggs with spinach and cherry tomatoes.
- Lunch: Quinoa salad with mixed vegetables (bell peppers, cucumber, carrots) and grilled chicken breast
- Dinner: Baked salmon with roasted sweet potatoes and steamed broccoli

Day 2:

- Breakfast: Greek yogurt parfait with mixed berries and granola
- Lunch: Turkey and avocado wrap with whole grain tortilla, lettuce, and tomato
- Dinner: Stir-fried tofu with mixed vegetables (broccoli, bell peppers, snap peas) served over brown rice

Day 3:

- Breakfast: Oatmeal topped with sliced banana, almonds, and a drizzle of honey

- Lunch: Spinach and feta stuffed chicken breast with quinoa and roasted Brussels sprouts
- Dinner: Shrimp and vegetable stir-fry with cauliflower rice

Day 4:

- Breakfast: Smoothie bowl with blended spinach, kale, banana, and protein powder topped with granola, sliced strawberries, and chia seeds
- Lunch: Chickpea and vegetable curry served with quinoa
- Dinner: Baked chicken thighs with roasted root vegetables (carrots, parsnips, and beets) and a side of steamed asparagus

Day 5:

- Breakfast: Whole grain pancakes topped with Greek yogurt and mixed berries
- Lunch: Turkey and black bean lettuce wraps with avocado, salsa, and a side of brown rice

- Dinner: Beef stir-fry with bok choy, mushrooms, and bell peppers served over cauliflower rice

Day 6:

- Breakfast: Egg muffins with spinach, mushrooms, and feta cheese
- Lunch: Lentil and vegetable soup with a side of whole grain bread
- Dinner: Grilled shrimp skewers with pineapple chunks and zucchini served with quinoa

Day 7:

- Breakfast: Overnight oats made with rolled oats, almond milk, chia seeds, and sliced peaches, topped with a dollop of almond butter.
- Lunch: Grilled vegetable and hummus wrap with whole grain tortilla, including grilled zucchini, bell peppers, and eggplant.
- Dinner: Baked tofu with roasted Brussels sprouts and a side of quinoa pilaf mixed with dried cranberries and sliced almonds.

Day 8:

- Breakfast: Whole grain toast with mashed avocado and poached eggs
- Lunch: Quinoa salad with roasted vegetables (such as bell peppers, zucchini, and cherry tomatoes) and grilled shrimp
- Dinner: Baked cod with lemon and herbs, served with steamed green beans and wild rice

Day 9:

- Breakfast: Smoothie made with spinach, kale, pineapple, banana, and coconut water
- Lunch: Turkey and vegetable stir-fry with snow peas, carrots, and broccoli served over brown rice
- Dinner: Lentil soup with a side of mixed green salad and whole grain bread

Day 10:

- Breakfast: Scrambled tofu with sautéed spinach, mushrooms, and onions, served with whole grain toast

- Lunch: Grilled chicken Caesar salad with romaine lettuce, cherry tomatoes, Parmesan cheese, and homemade Caesar dressing
- Dinner: Beef and broccoli stir-fry with a side of quinoa

Day 11:

- Breakfast: Greek yogurt with sliced banana, walnuts, and a drizzle of honey
- Lunch: Black bean and corn salad with diced tomatoes, avocado, and cilantro lime dressing
- Dinner: Baked turkey meatballs with marinara sauce, served over spaghetti squash

Day 12:

- Breakfast: Overnight chia seed pudding with almond milk, topped with mixed berries and shredded coconut
- Lunch: Salmon salad with mixed greens, cucumber, avocado, and balsamic vinaigrette
- Dinner: Vegetable and tofu curry served with quinoa

Day 13:

- Breakfast: Whole grain waffles topped with Greek yogurt and sliced strawberries
- Lunch: Chickpea and vegetable stir-fry with bell peppers, snap peas, and carrots served over couscous
- Dinner: Grilled shrimp tacos with cabbage slaw, avocado, and salsa, served in corn tortillas

Day 14:

- Breakfast: Breakfast burrito with scrambled eggs, black beans, diced bell peppers, and salsa wrapped in a whole grain tortilla
- Lunch: Quinoa and black bean stuffed bell peppers topped with melted cheese and served with a side salad
- Dinner: Baked chicken thighs with roasted sweet potatoes and steamed broccoli

Day 15:

- Breakfast: Smoothie bowl with blended acai, mixed berries, banana, and granola

- Lunch: Turkey and avocado wrap with spinach, tomato, and whole grain tortilla
- Dinner: Stir-fried tofu with mixed vegetables (such as broccoli, bell peppers, and snap peas) served over brown rice

Day 16:

- Breakfast: Oatmeal topped with sliced apple, almonds, and a drizzle of maple syrup
- Lunch: Spinach and feta stuffed chicken breast with quinoa and roasted Brussels sprouts
- Dinner: Shrimp and vegetable stir-fry with cauliflower rice

Day 17:

- Breakfast: Greek yogurt parfait with mixed berries and granola
- Lunch: Lentil and vegetable soup with a side of whole grain bread
- Dinner: Baked salmon with roasted root vegetables (carrots, parsnips, and beets) and steamed asparagus

Day 18:

- Breakfast: Egg muffins with spinach, mushrooms, and feta cheese
- Lunch: Grilled vegetable and hummus wrap with whole grain tortilla
- Dinner: Baked tofu with roasted Brussels sprouts and quinoa pilaf mixed with dried cranberries and sliced almonds

Day 19:

- Breakfast: Overnight oats with rolled oats, almond milk, chia seeds, and sliced peaches, topped with almond butter
- Lunch: Grilled shrimp skewers with pineapple chunks and zucchini served with quinoa
- Dinner: Beef stir-fry with bok choy, mushrooms, and bell peppers served over cauliflower rice.

Day 20:

- Breakfast: Smoothie made with spinach, kale, banana, and protein powder

- Lunch: Turkey and black bean lettuce wraps with avocado, salsa, and brown rice
- Dinner: Baked chicken thighs with roasted vegetables and a side of steamed green beans

Day 21:

- Breakfast: Whole grain toast with mashed avocado and poached eggs
- Lunch: Quinoa salad with mixed vegetables and grilled shrimp
- Dinner: Lentil soup with a side of mixed green salad and whole grain bread

Meal Prep Tips

1. Prep Ingredients in Advance:
   - Wash, chop, and portion out fruits and vegetables for easy grab-and-go options throughout the week.
   - Cook grains like quinoa, brown rice, and sweet potatoes in bulk to use in various meals.

2. Cook Proteins in Bulk:

- Grill or bake chicken breasts, salmon fillets, and tofu ahead of time to add to salads, wraps, or stir-fries.

3. Portion Control:

- Use portion control containers or simply divide your cooked meals into individual containers to avoid overeating.

4. Keep Snacks Ready:

- Prepare healthy snacks like sliced vegetables, hummus, Greek yogurt, or mixed nuts to curb cravings between meals.

5. Experiment with Different Cooking Methods:

- Try baking, grilling, steaming, or stir-frying your ingredients to add variety to your meals and flavors.

6. Incorporate a Variety of Foods:

- Include a mix of lean proteins, whole grains, healthy fats, and plenty of fruits and vegetables to ensure balanced nutrition.

7. Stay Hydrated:

- Drink plenty of water throughout the day to stay hydrated and support your metabolism.

11. CONCLUSION

Starting the Metabolic Confusion diet involves accepting a lifestyle shift rather than just picking up a new eating habit. Endomorph women have a different path since they have particular difficulties controlling their weight and metabolism. The information and resources included in this book are intended to provide you with the skills needed to effectively handle these obstacles.

Recognizing Metabolic Confusion: This diet's main focus is on adjusting calorie intake to avoid metabolic standstill, which improves weight reduction and metabolic health in general.

Personalization: There is no one-size-fits-all approach to nutrition and fitness. It is important to customize the Metabolic Confusion diet to each person's unique requirements, preferences, and reactions.

Combining Diet and Exercise: For endomorphs in particular, HIIT, weight training, and cardio should be included in addition to the nutritional component of Metabolic Confusion.

Mindful Eating and Emotional Control: Two essential elements of a successful diet plan are cultivating a positive connection with food and controlling emotional eating.

Overcoming Plateaus: Recognizing and overcoming plateaus in weight reduction by modifying lifestyle, nutrition, and activity choices.

Remind yourself as you go that achieving health and fitness is a lifelong, dynamic process. It's about incorporating long-lasting adjustments into your way of life.

Keep Up Your Knowledge: Never stop learning about diet, physical activity, and metabolic health. A strong tool for sustaining your health journey is knowledge.

Seek Support: Don't be afraid to ask for help from experts, communities, or support groups.

Be Kind and Patient with Yourself: Change takes time, and development may sometimes go slowly. Throughout the process, keep in mind to be gentle to yourself and patient.

Consider how you might advance in your health journey by continuing to develop and adapt in the future.

Frequent Health Check-ups: Make sure you schedule routine medical examinations and discussions with specialists.

Lifelong Learning: Remain receptive to fresh findings and innovations in the fitness and nutrition sectors.

Motivating Others: Disseminate your experiences and insights to others. Someone else could be motivated and inspired by your experience.

A novel and flexible strategy for maintaining metabolic health and controlling weight is provided by the Metabolic Confusion diet. Through comprehension and implementation of the concepts presented in this book, you might potentially improve your physical well-being and develop a more profound understanding of your body and its requirements. Accept this path as a chance for development, well-being, and health.

Recall that your adventure does not finish with the publication of this book. You're starting a new chapter in your life, one in which you have more knowledge and authority to choose what's best for your health and wellbeing. Proceed with forward motion, maintain your curiosity, and allow your path to well-being to develop further.